Postpartum Action Manual

How to Provide Comfort, Encouragement, and Guidance to New Families

A Pragmatic Approach to Reach and Teach Peer Leaders

Jane I. Honikman, M.S.

Disclaimer: The information contained in this publication is advisory only and is not intended to replace sound clinical judgment or individualized patient care. The author disclaims all warranties, whether expressed or implied, including any warranty as the quality, accuracy, safety, or suitability of this information for any particular purpose.

ISBN 978-0692459461

Printed in the United States of America

Cover design and book layout: Dowitcher Designs

To obtain copies of this book, please visit: www.janehonikman.com

This book is dedicated to all the past, present, and future volunteers at
Postpartum Education for Parents (PEP) and
Postpartum Support International (PSI).

In appreciation to those who provide comfort, encouragement,
and guidance to new families.

Table of Contents

Preface 7

Foreword 9

Introduction 13

How to Use This Manual 15

Sessions

1 Opening: Introductions and Expectations 17

2 Perceptions of Depression 19

3 Postpartum Depression (PPD) 21

4 How to Communicate with Parents Experiencing PPD Signs and Symptoms ... 25

5 The Steps to Wellness 29

6 Creating an Action Plan 31

7 Building a Supportive Community 33

8 Conclusion, Wrap Up, and Evaluation 35

Handouts 37

Sources 47

Preface

More than fifty years ago, Jane and I met, and we began a shared journey that continues to amaze me. She could think on her feet and had vision. She also had much to teach me, and fortunately, I was open and willing to learn. Jane's insights and her determination have changed me profoundly, but more importantly, she has changed the lives of parents and families around the world. For more than four decades, she has been taking abstract ideas, defining real world problems, and building vibrant organizations to deal with those problems. As a result, I have always felt driven to support her as she has tried to take each next step. It has always been exciting for me to gain understanding of her latest idea, and while reading her latest work, I had another "aha" moment. In her Forward for *Postpartum Action Manual,* I saw the issue from a new vantage point. And what a significant perspective it is. She has found the missing piece in a puzzle.

So, what is this missing piece? Jane has identified one of the root explanations of why Postpartum Education for Parents (PEP) has not spread beyond Santa Barbara. Until there are trained peer support parent volunteers in every community, the concept of easing the adjustment to parenthood cannot be implemented organically. This is a profound idea. It is the essence of a movement for millions of people around the world, without taxing them financially. That easing of transitional stress will provide many rewards to each community, not the least of which will be improved mental health and all the benefits that will flow from it. In a world that depends on evidence-based solutions, we need look no further than PEP. Now the world needs action toward spreading Jane's ideas.

Terry Honikman
Santa Barbara, California

Foreword

When a newborn baby has arrived, either by adoption or birth, the word *postpartum* refers to that stage in human development. It is correct to state, "I am *postpartum*. I've just had a baby."

The word *postpartum* is an adjective. It describes a noun. If you are not feeling like yourself after the arrival of your baby, then it may be accurate to say, "I have *postpartum* blues or depression." It is not correct to state, "I have *postpartum*." If you do not feel depressed, it is not correct to say, "I am not *postpartum*." The word *postpartum* is not a noun.

I have a personal connection to the use, misuse, and confusion around the usage of the word *postpartum*. I feel a sense of responsibility to explain the evolution of this adjective in our vernacular. It began in the 1970s.

When my friends and I founded Postpartum Education for Parents (PEP), we took a risk. The words antenatal, prenatal and postnatal were used by the childbirth education and breastfeeding groups. We wanted to emphasize the experience after birth and joked about naming our new organization "Afterbirth." Postpartum was the perfect word and it garnered attention because it was unique. An article I wrote in 1977 presents the background to why and how I got involved in postpartum mental health and emotional support. It is called "My Onset of Parenthood."

It was 2 AM and Stephen would not stop crying. He was four days old and creating an increasingly difficult situation for his unskilled, new parents. If only we could go back to the hospital, I wished. It was so organized and peaceful there. My attempts to calm him and my urgent desire for some sleep were being ruined by his incessant crying. In total frustration, I placed him on the floor next to the rocking chair (where we had been trying to act out the picture-perfect mother-and-child scene) and I ran from his room in tears. I met his equally distraught father in the hallway and sobbed, "I don't know what to do with him, you take care of him."

> *"Is he sick, shall we call the doctor?"*
>
> *"I don't think so, besides, we can't bother him at this hour."*
>
> *"Is he hungry?"*
>
> *"I don't know, I just nursed him." And so it went.*

It has been five and a half years since we experienced that and many other similar scenes as first time parents. Somehow, through trial and error, crisis and pleasure, we managed to survive the new roles which we had created for ourselves. We discovered, to our dismay, that no matter how well planned our pregnancy had been, or how well we had prepared for childbirth, the onset of parenthood generated a wave of emotional ripples that we had not anticipated.

At times I wondered, did it have to be this bad, as I appeared all smiles on the outside and seethed with tension on the inside. Wasn't anyone else feeling the same distress, pretending it was so simple when it felt impossible? It took time for us to find other couples who were willing to admit that they too were having difficulties adjusting to their new roles as parents, with our changed lifestyles. When we could talk about it, we agreed that parenting required skills which were acquired through experience or training. The magical instinct that guided new parents turned out to be only a myth. Just as we had learned that the stork had not brought our babies, we had discovered that the bird of paradise could not help with their raising. But what could be done for other families? How could those couples with experience help new parents?

This question kept challenging me. Fortunately, I met other parents who were also seeking an answer to this question. In January 1976, I helped in the formulation of a new community organization called Postpartum Education for Parents, or PEP. Our group was designed to carry on where childbirth education left off, with the arrival of the baby. The goal was to ease the adjustment of the developing family by providing emotional support through trained parent volunteers. We planned to offer two free services, a 24 hour, 7 day per week Warm Line and Parent Discussion Groups. The Warm Line would use an answering service to allow the volunteers to work from their own homes. The concept of a "warm" in contrast to a "hot" line was chosen to encourage a wide scope of calls. Our intent was to appear as nonthreatening as possible so that parents who could not call a stress line would feel comfortable with the PEP Warm Line. Whenever a medical or psychological problem would arise, the volunteers would be trained to refer the parent to a specific agency, a doctor, or other professional. Our goal was to provide nonjudgmental environments, on the phone or in a group setting, where parents could discuss their concerns and questions, both negative and positive, about parenthood. The sharing of ideas would increase the parents' sense of confidence and allow them to make their own decisions regarding their families.

To begin with we needed to have the backing of the community, especially those in the health professions. Our first support came from the childbirth educators of Santa Barbara and then from the Santa Barbara Pediatric Society. In no way did we want to interfere with the medical profession, instead we wanted to assist the services which already existed. We impressed the child psychiatrist at the Santa Barbara County Department of Mental Health, and he secured the underwriting of our printing costs for up to $350. This gave us the necessary incentive to finish the writing of a Reference Guide designed to assist training our volunteers and to create a PEP brochure. An advisory board was established with representatives from obstetrics-gynecology, pediatrics, psychology-counseling, OB nursing, childbirth education, and psychiatry. With their liaison into the community sectors from which they came, we were able to continue to build our reputation.

As of July 1, 1977, PEP is a reality and we have fourteen trained parent volunteers. The ideal volunteer is a parent who has an understanding of his or her own feelings and experiences relating to that role. She or he must be caring, be able to relate to, and communicate with other people. After completing a written application, the volunteer is interviewed and then attends two all day training sessions. These workshops are intended to provide the parents with the skills necessary for responding objectively and compassionately to Warm Line calls. We are able to offer the Warm Line because of a $500 Research and Projects Grant from the American Association of University Women's Education Foundation.

The type of phone calls we receive reflect the need for PEP. "What do you do with a non-participating father?" "My baby is two months old and seems unusually fussy." "Is it common to feel less interested in sex while I'm nursing?" In response, we listen objectively, ask many questions, offer suggestions, and encourage the parents to consider the alternatives available to answer their questions. We make it clear that there are few concrete rules to follow. If there is the slightest hint of the need for medication or other assistance, we refer the parents to the proper resource in Santa Barbara. A follow-up call is made within the next few days to offer further assistance and support. An invitation to attend a parents' discussion group is always extended. We adhere to strict confidentiality.

The satisfaction I feel from helping to organize PEP is deep. To know that my past frustrations and sense of isolation are easing some of that for other new parents is satisfying. My experiences are still fresh in my mind as I respond to a tired parent's call. "Yes, I know exactly what you must be feeling right now, let's talk about it."

"My Onset of Parenthood" is the foundation of my involvement in the parental mental health movement. There is no mention of postpartum depression in my story because it was an unknown topic when PEP was established. It is the journey from starting PEP to founding Postpartum Support International (PSI) in 1987 that led me to write this *Manual*. For five years after founding PEP there was national publicity and inquiries from journalists. One in particular was researching postpartum depression. Her call changed my life and the way that the adjective, postpartum, would change as well.

Introduction

This *Postpartum Action Manual* is designed to promote community conversations about new family emotional support. My goal is to reach and teach parents to be peer leaders. This is accomplished through an interactive workshop format described in this *Manual*. It combines information contained in my previous publications, *Community Support for New Families* and *I'm Listening*. My book *Community Support for New Families* is designed as a "fill-in-the-blank" workbook. Its companion guide, *I'm Listening*, is written in a narrative format. *Postpartum Action Manual* combines these and gives direction on how to facilitate conversations, ask questions, probe for answers, discuss, encourage interaction, and learn how to implement suggested actions, and change in a community. Postpartum Action workshops provide time to practice active listening skills through role playing. Rather than listening to lectures that are one-sided it is time to engage with one another, discover one's own motivations, question our egos, reach out, recruit, and train others.

My focus is on mental wellbeing. I want participants to feel comfortable about the topic of depression and learn and practice how to empower parents, their families, and others. Scientific research on parental mental illness continues to search for answers. Lectures on the latest research are presented at conferences. Papers are published in journals that may be read but primarily sit on shelves. Some puzzling questions are solved and stimulating discussions spin. Meanwhile new families continue to struggle with what they are experiencing, wondering what is normal and what is not. There are huge gulfs between promoting wellness, prevention of illness, and early intervention when it is required. I believe experienced parent activists who are willing to get involved with the transition to parenthood are the missing link.

The content of this *Manual* compiles my decades of hands-on experience supporting new parents and grandparents and my determination to advocate for them. It evolved from my commonsense approach to life in general. It is logical and simple, but based on scientific research about the importance and power of social support. It is both pragmatic and heartfelt.

This *Postpartum Action Manual* is created for individuals who identify themselves as committed to confronting the stigma of mental illness and mythology surrounding new parenthood. I want to recruit and inspire participants who are interested in challenging the status quo of separating mental health from physical health. These individuals should be willing to find the current gaps in social and medical services and improve community resources for new parents. We need the courage to challenge current health care practices, approaches, and assumptions. Why are we afraid to ask ourselves and others key questions regarding family history of mental illness, secrets, and traumas? Why do we divide conception, birth, and human development into separate categories? What makes us so afraid of strange thoughts and behaviors? How can we become more empathetic and attentive to the needs of others? How do we make healthier communities? It requires social action.

Social action requires being able to question the status quo, explore options, make inquiries about existing services, and envision alternatives. My *Postpartum Action Manual* is the result of my curiosity, tenacity, and luck.

I desire change and have had some success. For example, I read about the international humanitarian organization CARE (Cooperative for Assistance and Relief Everywhere, Inc.) in the 2010 book *Half the Sky* by Nicholas Kristof and Sheryl WuDunn. CARE is a leader in the fight against global poverty. In 2011, I attended my first CARE USA Conference held in Washington, DC. It was an impressive gathering of political and social luminaries. The CARE Mission is to empower women and girls. The organization is successful and effective. During the conference, I participated in a workshop on maternal health which, while informative, did not mention mental health. I boldly asked about CARE's policy regarding maternal depression. There was silence from the panelists, and applause from the audience. The lack of an affirmative response did not deter me. I approached a board member and asked the question again. She handed me her card and promised to find an answer. I was introduced to the Senior Director of Health Programs at CARE USA headquarters in Atlanta, Georgia. I learned about their early childhood development (ECD) program and their 5 X 5 model that crosses five domains; nutrition, health, development, protection, and safety, with five levels; the child, parents, childcare setting, community, and region/country. I was told about their "Essential Package" strategy and tool kit they were developing that would include postpartum depression. My timing was perfect!

The questions I asked led to *I'm Listening* being adapted into the *CARE Facilitator's Training Guide How to Help Families Cope with Postpartum Depression* for use at one of their projects in Bangladesh. CARE's "Window of Opportunity" program is named for the key time of pregnancy through age two for the prevention of malnutrition. Their strategy includes mother-to-mother support groups to address maternal depression and breastfeeding. The Guide was published in March 2012 by CARE for use by the Nutrition Plus team. They tested an intervention where community nutrition counselors were taught to deliver basic psycho-social support services to women and their familiess. I participated in a webinar when their results were presented one year later at the CARE Health Equity Unit meeting. The title of the presentation was "Where there is no psychologist/psychiatrist: How to help families cope with postpartum depression in Bangladesh." Needless to say, I was overjoyed by the outcome of my initial action. I gratefully acknowledge the CARE publication and its use in Bangladesh.

This *Postpartum Action Manual* is a refinement of what I learned from CARE's practical and common-sense approach to working with families in a developing country. Even in developed countries there is a chasm between what parents need and what professionals offer. It is my hope that by using this *Postpartum Action Manual* we can work together and go beyond talk, fill the gap to make postpartum action happen in villages, towns, and cities around the globe.

My vision is to have a parent support network in every community in the world. It is based on the success of Postpartum Education for Parents (PEP). I believe that with a hands-on, interactive approach we can advance this dream and have a positive impact on new parents, grandparents, and their children.

How to Use This Manual

This *Manual* is designed to be used to lead and facilitate an interactive workshop. The content is divided into eight topic sessions. Icons are used throughout the book to denote when the facilitator should read out loud, lead an activity, or note a key point.

The recommended time required for the workshop is eight hours. There are suggested times for each session, however, they are approximate. It will depend on the number of participants and how engaged they are with specific topics. The expectation is for a highly active learning process. A nutrition break up to an hour long should be provided after Session 4. Small breaks and refreshments should be provided between sessions as needed.

Sessions:

1 Opening: Introductions and Expectations

2 Perceptions of Depression

3 Postpartum Depression (PPD)

4 How to Communicate with Parents Experiencing PPD Signs and Symptoms

5 The Steps to Wellness

6 Creating an Action Plan

7 Building a Supportive Community

8 Conclusion, Wrap Up, and Evaluation

Workshop Preparation:

All participants will need pens or pencils for this workshop. The handouts at the back of the manual will be used by the participants for taking notes. Depending upon the number of participants and the size of the room, large poster paper, markers, and an easel may be needed.

Workshop Mood:

The leader's role is as a facilitator throughout the learning process. The topics are sensitive and challenging to talk about. It is important to explain that while the content may produce emotional reactions, the workshop mood should be relaxed and comfortable. Face-to-face interaction requires that the seating arrangement be in one or more circles depending upon the number of participants and size of the room.

Workshop Goals:

1. To reach and teach parents to be peer leaders

2. To have participants feel comfortable about the topic of depression

3. To learn and practice how to empower parents, their families, and others

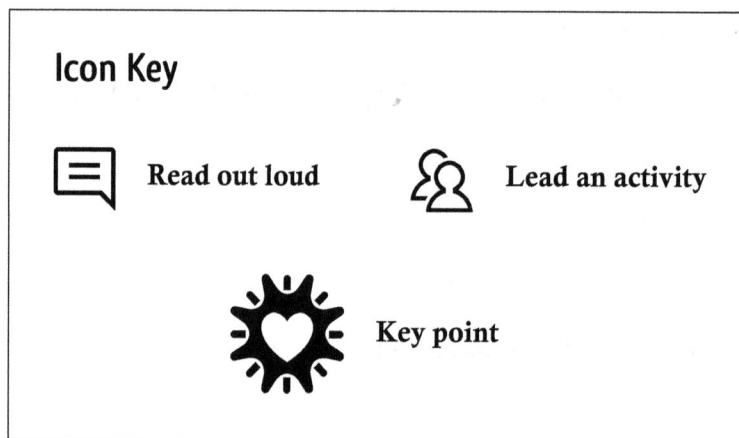

Icon Key

Read out loud   Lead an activity

Key point

SESSION 1
Opening: Introductions and Expectations

Session 1 has four steps. It should take approximately 30 minutes. It is designed to make the participants feel welcome and comfortable, and to establish a friendly, open atmosphere of trust. The success of this workshop is based on dialogue and interaction among the participants. As Leader, you are responsible for setting this mood.

Step 1

Read out loud from the author Jane Honikman: This Postpartum Action workshop is designed to promote community conversations about new family emotional support. The goal is to reach and teach parents to be peer leaders. Postpartum Action workshops provide time to practice active listening skills through role playing. The focus is on mental wellbeing. I want participants to feel comfortable about the topic of depression and learn and practice how to empower parents, their families, and others. New families continue to struggle with what they are experiencing, wondering what is normal and what is not. I believe experienced parent activists who are willing to get involved with the transition to parenthood are the missing link. This workshop is created for individuals who identify themselves as committed to confronting the stigma of mental illness and mythology surrounding new parenthood. I want to recruit and inspire participants who are interested in challenging the status quo of separating mental health from physical health. It requires social action. My vision is to have a postpartum parent support network in every community in the world.

Step 2

Introduce yourself and welcome all the participants to the workshop. Have all the participants introduce themselves by their name and the community where they work and live.

Step 3

Read out loud: This workshop is intended to teach you to provide postpartum emotional support to parents and family members.

Postpartum denotes the period from arrival through the first year of life of a baby.

By the end of this workshop you will have:

1. Learned about postpartum depression (PPD)

2. Learned how to provide quality, personalized support for women and men experiencing PPD

3. Learned the *Steps to Wellness* that can help empower people to help themselves

4. Learned how to help individuals create a plan of action to help them assess their strengths and needs

5. Learned how to build a supportive community for families experiencing PPD

Step 4

Lead the following ice breaker. This exercise helps set the tone of the workshop as friendly and informal.

Names and adjectives:

Ask the participants to think of an adjective to describe themselves. The adjective must start with the same letter as their name, for instance, "I'm Chris and I'm creative." or, "I'm Amy and I'm amazing." As they say this, they can also mime an action that describes the adjective.

SESSION 2
Perceptions of Depression

Session 2 has two steps. Allow about 30 minutes. It is designed to promote discussion among the participants about their own points of view about depression. The conversational format encourages honesty about current beliefs.

Step 1

Read out loud: I will now read a story, please listen carefully. This is a case vignette on depression adapted from a research study on cultural dimensions of depression in Bangladesh.

A new mother complains of different troubles right after having her baby. Troubles, such as headache, pain in the stomach, general weakness of the body, and tiredness. She has not been doing her work as well as she usually does. She finds it difficult to sleep. In addition, she is worried about problems she faces (money, children, housing) and is irritable with close relatives and friends. She cannot relax or enjoy herself properly.

The following discussion is about the participants' points of view, perceptions, and perspectives. The role of the facilitator is to be an active listener and encourage discussion as needed. The participants must listen carefully to each other throughout this process. Points of view reflect one's own experience, education, and training.

Step 2

Hold a focus group discussion. Listen to the discussions and probe, if needed.

1. What do you think about what was read?

2. What do you think are the causes of her situation?

3. Does this mother have a problem or an illness?

4. If she has a problem, what would you call it? Is it an illness, why?

5. Is this condition physical, mental, both, or social?

6. What can be done about her situation?

7. What suggestions do you have for providing treatment, if needed?

8. What do you think works best—prevention or cure?

9. Do you think that this problem can be prevented and how?

10. What are the most important results you think she would receive from a treatment?

11. If left untreated, will her situation get worse?

12. Do you think that her problems are harmful to herself, the baby, her family, or the community?

13. How do you think this problem might impact the baby's father?

14. What impact will there be on other family members?

15. How capable do you think she will be at work?

16. Who do you think suffers the most from this condition?

Session 3
Postpartum Depression (PPD)

Session 3 has six steps and is designed to delve into the details about the who, why, what of postpartum depression, and how to be supportive. This section puts everyone on the same knowledge level and takes about one hour.
Pass out Handout 1.

Step 1

Read out loud: What is Postpartum Depression (PPD)?

Depression is characterized by low mood, sadness, and loss of interest in daily activities that persist for long periods of time. Anxiety is part of depression.

The term **postpartum** describes the first year after the arrival of a baby.

Postpartum depression (PPD) is depression that occurs for up to a year after the arrival or loss of a baby. A parent suffering from PPD may experience one or a combination of symptoms, each ranging from mild to severe.

Fathers can also be depressed. All discussions need to include the baby's father as well as the relationship of the couple. Grandparents' experiences are important too and should be included.

Step 2

Ask the participants to read aloud, one at a time, the bulleted symptoms in Handout 1. Ask for comments and if they have additional words they'd like to add to the list.

Step 3

Read out loud: Additionally a new parent may experience the following:

- Have trouble sleeping when the baby sleeps (more than the lack of sleep new parents usually experience).

- Feel numb or disconnected from the baby.

- Have scary or negative thoughts about the baby, such as thinking someone will take the baby away or hurt the baby.

21

- Worry that they will hurt the baby.

- Feel guilty about not being a good parent, or ashamed that she or he cannot care for the baby.

Emphasize this point! When these symptoms occur within the first year after the arrival of the baby, and last for more than a week or two at a time, this is postpartum depression. Key aspects are onset, intensity, and duration.

Step 4

Read out loud: Who gets PPD?

Being a mom or dad is hard. For some, the journey to becoming a parent is really hard too. Often, trying to get pregnant, being pregnant, or the birth of the baby can increase the risk for depression. Adoptive parents can also get PPD.

Depression is a common problem during and after pregnancy. Approximately 10% of new mothers and fathers have postpartum depression (PPD).

PPD can affect any woman: women with easy or problematic pregnancies, easy or traumatic deliveries, young or old mothers, first-time mothers and those with one or more children, and any woman regardless of income, race, ethnicity, culture, or education. The research is not as clear for men.

Step 5

Read out loud: Why does it happen?

During the time immediately after birth, the woman's body undergoes rapid hormonal changes to adjust for no longer needing to support a baby. It is thought that these hormone changes can make women more vulnerable to depression. Additionally, poverty, family problems, lack of support, and other daily stressors can contribute to the challenges of the postpartum period and increase the risk of depression. The same can be said for fathers and grandparents.

Individuals with a family and/or personal history of depression are most at risk for PPD. Also, women who experienced PPD with one child are more likely to suffer it with subsequent births.

Many women and men feel especially guilty about having depressive feelings at a time when they believe they should be happy. They may be reluctant to discuss their symptoms or their negative feelings toward the child.

Other factors may play a role in postpartum depression:

- Anxiety or negative feelings about the pregnancy

- Stress from changes in work and home routines

- An unrealistic need to be a perfect parent

- Difficult family relationships

Parents need support and encouragement after they welcome a child into their life.

Step 6

Read out loud: How can you support a parent experiencing postpartum depression?

Women need to be nurtured to recover from pregnancy and childbirth. The first and most important thing you can do to help a parent who is suffering from depression is to nurture her/him. You essentially need to provide "nurturing" to the parents. The act of "nurturing" may even prevent an onset of depression. Fathers must also be acknowledged in their role. Support new parents by offering to provide food, help around the house, run errands, and care for the baby. A family without healthy parents will not be a healthy family.

It is important to identify those who are suffering more severe symptoms, including suicidal or homicidal thoughts, and immediately refer them to the appropriate professionals.

Notes

SESSION 4
How to Communicate with Parents Experiencing PPD Signs and Symptoms

Session 4 has five steps and requires about an hour to complete. It includes role playing followed by discussions. **Pass out Handout 2.** At the end of this session allow the participants a nutrition break up to an hour long. This is an opportunity to build relationships among the attendees.

Step 1

Read out loud: A new parent is someone who has given birth (or adopted) in the past year. They are considered "new" after the arrival of each child. Each new baby makes a woman a new mother and a man a new father.

There are **three universal needs** of parents, no matter who they are or where they live:

1. A companion or spokesperson through pregnancy, delivery, and the postpartum year.

2. Supportive and trained professionals.

3. A time and a place to share pregnancy, birth, and postpartum experiences.

All families deserve these fundamentals of care and concern, but these needs are frequently unmet. Unfulfilled expectations about being emotionally and physically supported can lead to stress and distress. As a support person listening to concerns, you have an opportunity to fulfill some expectations and at least some needs. It is important that parents also find someone else to listen to them such as their own parents, in-laws, other relatives, neighbors, or friends. This requires active listening so the parents will feel heard and understood.

Step 2

Ask the participants to read aloud, one at a time, the bulleted points in Handout 2.

Key points of active listening and effective questioning:

*   Use body language to show interest and understanding. In most cultures this will include nodding the head and turning the body to face the person speaking.

- Use facial expressions to show interest and reflect on what is being said. This may include looking directly at the person speaking, although in some cultures such direct eye contact may not be appropriate until some trust has been established.

- Listen to how things are said by paying attention to a speaker's body language and tone of voice.

- Ask questions to show a desire to understand.

- Summarize and rephrase the discussions to check on an understanding of what has been said and ask for feedback.

- Leave time for silence.

- Know the facts about the topic.

- Be informative, but don't lecture.

- Never judge, no matter what the parent tells you.

- Give people time to come up with their own ideas.

- Stand or sit at the same level as the speaker.

- Ask open-ended questions–for example, using the six key 'helper' questions (Why? What? When? Where? Who? and How?).

- Ask probing questions by following up people's answers with further questions that look deeper into the issue; continually asking, 'But why…?' is useful for doing this.

- Ask clarifying questions to ensure they have been understood, which can be done by rewording a previous question.

- Ask questions about personal points of view by asking how people feel and not just about what they know.

Step 3

Read out loud: When establishing a relationship of trust with a new parent your voice needs to convey a sense of validation (that you value what the parent is sharing with you), reassurance, warmth, and hope. Read out loud, one participant at a time, the list of questions on the back of Handout 2.

Step 4

Tell the participants that they will now practice establishing trust. Have them split into pairs to role play. Have the participants practice **active listening and effective questioning.** One participant should play the role of the mother/father and the other participant should play the role of the supportive person and then the pair should switch roles. Have the participant role playing the parent act like they are experiencing symptoms of PPD. Have the participants playing the supportive part pay attention to their body language when role playing. The supportive person needs to establish that they are "warm" and "caring" individuals. After both participants have had the chance to role play each part, have them provide feedback to each other on their active listening and effective questioning skills. Step 4 should take approximately 10-15 minutes.

Listen carefully to the role play exercise and monitor the time it is taking. Be mindful that the supportive person must not dominate with his or her own personal stories.

Step 5

Tell the participants that it is always important to debrief participants after a role play.

Lead a group discussion about how this practice felt. Ask the participants what it felt like for them to role play the part of the parent. Ask whether or not they felt supported. Role plays can bring up a lot of emotions. People might be reminded of their own painful experiences or the experiences of family or friends. Be aware of that and provide plenty of time for discussion.

Notes

SESSION 5
The Steps to Wellness

Session 5 has three steps and includes an activity that visually emphasizes components of good mental health care. The content is based on *Steps to Wellness* and continues into session 6. **Pass out Handout 3.**

Step 1

Read out loud: There are three important messages that every parent should hear. They are:

1. You are not alone.

2. You are not to blame for what you are feeling.

3. You will be well and feel like yourself again.

Our next activity involves completing a sun diagram on Handout 3. This tool will identify actions that new parents, family members, and friends can take to help cope with PPD.

Step 2

Tell the participants to follow these steps for the sun diagram activity:

1. Write actions that parents could do that would help them cope with PPD on the rays of the sun diagram.

2. Discuss in pairs or as a group all the possible actions that could be taken to help cope with PPD.

3. Encourage the participants to keep going until they have identified all of the possible actions they can think of. As a group, discuss what the diagram shows. For example, how many actions are there? Which actions are easier or harder for parents to do?

Step 3

Tell the participants to read *Steps to Wellness* on the back of Handout 3. Review the list of these potential actions if they were not discussed during the activity in Step 2 in pairs, small groups, or as a whole.

Steps to Wellness:

Education about PPD: It is important that everyone knows about the onset, intensity, and duration of the signs and symptoms of PPD.

Sleep: Recovery depends on quality of sleep. Sleep can heal the body and mind. Someone who is not sleeping well may be suffering from depression or anxiety.

Eating nutritious food: If parents are not eating well, no one will thrive—including the baby.

Exercise and time for oneself: To be healthy the body requires a balance of sleep, food, and movement.

Nonjudgmental listening from others: New parents need to talk about their journey through pregnancy, birth or the adoption process, and parenthood.

Emotional support from others: New parents need supportive and caring people with whom to share and be heard.

Practical support from others: Parents need help.

Steps to Wellness **was originally designed for use over the telephone. Callers were asked to write down the key points listed above as each was explained by the listener. The caller was asked to review the list and make a plan of action before the conversation was concluded. This sun diagram activity can be used during a home visit or in a support group.**

SESSION 6
Creating an Action Plan

Session 6 is designed to practice "what can be done next" through four steps with role playing exercises and requires up to an hour to complete. **Continue to use Handout 3.**

Step 1

Read out loud: The Trials of Improved Practice is a procedure that comes from the Food and Agriculture Organization of the United Nations. It consists of a series of visits in which a support person and a participant analyze current practices. They discuss what could be improved and together they reach an agreement. After a trial period they then assess the experience. The support person gives feedback to the parents on their practices, what they're doing well and areas they might improve. The support person can give several relevant suggestions of actions to try for a period of time. These suggestions are discussed thoroughly and the parent selects ones to try during the next visit or phone call. The support person learns what and how the mother or father did and how she or he felt about the trial experience; what was easy and difficult, and if they discussed the new behaviors with anyone else.

Step 2

Read out loud: Helping someone create a personal plan of action begins with having a parent acknowledge his or her present state of health and how to improve it.

Refer to **Handout 3** passed out in Session 5. Review the *Steps to Wellness* and the sun diagram activity. The parents' responses to each step will assist in making an action plan.

Step 3

Tell the participants that they will now practice establishing trust. Have them split into pairs to role play making a plan of actions listed on the back of Handout 3. Continue working in small groups or in pairs. Now let's make a plan of actions based on answers to what is listed.

- How can you get more sleep?

- How is your appetite?

- Who can you ask for help?

- Who can you talk to about what you are experiencing?

Step 4

Read out loud: What will be the follow-up to the action plan? It is important to discuss working through obstacles to steps to wellness. Consider the following four key points.

1. What were the challenges for the parents and the support person?

2. Who had the most power?

3. What might happen next?

4. What follow-up will happen and by whom?

Are there any other barriers to discuss?

SESSION 7
Building a Supportive Community

Session 7 has three steps and is designed to look into the future based on an activity called "vision diagramming." It includes drawing, discussing, sharing, and using one's imagination. The time for this Session will depend upon the pace of the workshop. **Do not** neglect or eliminate this important concluding topic. **Handout 4 is passed out.**

Step 1

Read out loud: The information in Handout 4 comes from the community self-help movement of the 1990s. Peer support occurs when people provide knowledge, experience, emotional, social, or practical help to each other. Peer support not only decreases isolation, but it also offers an atmosphere of common purpose for learning to cope.

Peer support should strive to:

- Address the needs of at-risk populations.
  (women of reproductive age, parents-to-be, new parents)

- Confront social isolation.

- Serve as new sources of social support during short-term crises and life transitions.

- Promote coping skills and self-esteem.

- Provide positive role models.

- Display benefits of helping others.

- Meet needs of underserved portions of the population.

- Facilitate referrals to professionals when necessary.

- Enhance social ties to serve as a buffer to stress.

- Help people cope with stress and adversity.

- Educate professionals about gaps and problems in service delivery.

- Assist in development of needed programming for communities.

- Promote social action and funding needs.

- Promote new collaboration between self-help and professional communities.

Step 2

Read out loud: Our final activity is called a vision diagram. It gives us a chance to think and picture a positive future for one's community. This tool is used when people are working together to identify new services and resources.

A vision diagram helps to:

- Imagine a positive future – a vision – where new parents and their families receive support.

- Identify activities and resources that will help achieve this vision.

- Identify who might be involved in providing these activities and resources.

- Identify possible challenges in bringing about the vision.

- Discuss how to solve these challenges.

It is important that participants feel relaxed in this exercise and that they take the time to imagine a very positive future. Encourage participants to remember the role of peer support.

Step 3

Create a vision diagram. The following activity can be done in a variety of ways based on the number of participants and size of the room. It can work in small groups or as a whole. Use the back of Handout 4 or a large piece of paper on an easel. The following are key points:

1. Think about the current situation for new families in your community.

2. What support do new parents receive?

3. Imagine a future in which new parents and families are fully supported.

4. What would your role in this vision of the future be? What other roles might exist?

Have participants share their pictures with each other in small groups of three or four. Bring the group back together as a whole to share visions.

Session 8
Conclusion, Wrap Up, and Evaluation

Session 8 is designed to give the facilitator feedback. The four hours allocated for the workshop may be up, but **do not** neglect or eliminate this important opportunity to evaluate the participants' experience. **Pass out Handout 5.**

It is important to allow time for concluding and evaluating the workshop. This will require careful planning and use of time by the facilitator.

Ask the participants to review the goals and objectives listed on Handout 5 and write their feedback.

Workshop Goals:

1. To reach and teach parents to be peer leaders

2. To have participants feel comfortable about the topic of depression

3. To learn and practice how to empower parents, their families, and others

Workshop Objectives:

1. Learned about postpartum depression (PPD)

2. Learned how to provide quality, personalized support for women and men experiencing PPD

3. Learned the *Steps to Wellness* that can help empower people to help themselves

4. Learned how to help individuals create a plan of action to help them assess their strengths and needs

5. Learned how to build a supportive community for families experiencing PPD

Notes

Handout 1

Depression is characterized by low mood, sadness, and loss of interest in daily activities that persist for long periods of time. Anxiety is part of depression.

The term **postpartum** describes the first year after the arrival of a baby.

Postpartum depression (PPD) is depression that occurs for up to a year after the arrival or loss of a baby. A parent suffering from PPD may experience one or a combination of symptoms, each ranging from mild to severe.

- A low or sad mood
- Loss of interest in fun activities
- Feelings of worthlessness, shame, or guilt
- Thoughts that life is not worth living
- Exhaustion, insomnia
- Anxiety, tension, panic, fearfulness
- Irritability
- Hopelessness, tearfulness
- Poor concentration, memory loss
- Rapid mood swings
- Obsessions, frightening recurring thoughts
- Lack of enthusiasm
- Self-doubt, low self-esteem
- Eating disturbances, loss of appetite, eating too much
- Feeling distance/removed from or lack of love for baby and/or partner
- Thoughts of harming self and/or baby
- Isolation
- Agitation

Additionally, a new parent may:

- Have trouble sleeping when the baby sleeps (more than the lack of sleep new parents usually experience).

- Feel numb or disconnected from the baby.

- Have scary or negative thoughts about the baby, such as thinking someone will take the baby away or hurt the baby.

- Worry that they will hurt the baby.

- Feel guilty about not being a good parent, or ashamed that she or he cannot care for the baby.

When these symptoms occur within the first year after the arrival of the baby, and last for more than a week or two at a time, this is postpartum depression. Key aspects are onset, intensity, and duration. Parents may make a general statement about "not feeling like myself" or others may observe a mother or father as "not like they usually are."

Handout 2

Key points of active listening and effective questioning:

- Use body language to show interest and understanding. In most cultures this will include nodding the head and turning the body to face the person speaking.

- Use facial expressions to show interest and reflect on what is being said. This may include looking directly at the person speaking, although in some cultures such direct eye contact may not be appropriate until some trust has been established.

- Listen to how things are said by paying attention to a speaker's body language and tone of voice.

- Ask questions to show a desire to understand.

- Summarize and rephrase the discussions to check on an understanding of what has been said and ask for feedback.

- Leave time for silence.

- Know the facts about the topic.

- Be informative, but don't lecture.

- Never judge, no matter what the parent tells you.

- Give people time to come up with their own ideas.

- Stand or sit at the same level as the speaker.

- Ask open-ended questions – for example, using the six key 'helper' questions (Why? What? When? Where? Who? and How?).

- Ask probing questions by following up people's answers with further questions that look deeper into the issue; continually asking, 'But why...?' is useful for doing this.

- Ask clarifying questions to ensure they have been understood, which can be done by rewording a previous question.

- Ask questions about personal points of view by asking how people feel and not just about what they know.

Once trust has been established, the following statements or questions are appropriate to say or ask new parents:

1. Congratulations on the arrival of your child.

2. How old is your child now?

3. Parenthood is a unique and special role to play in life.

4. I am here to support you.

5. How was the pregnancy or adoption process?

6. How was the birth of your child?

7. What is it like for you to be a new parent or a parent again?

8. How are you feeling emotionally after the arrival of your baby? Are you feeling different than what you typically feel like?

9. If the mother or father states she or he has been experiencing symptoms of PPD ask, "When did you first notice you weren't feeling like yourself?" Additionally, ask the parent, "Have you told anyone else how you are feeling?"

10. What are you doing to take care of yourself?

11. Can you sleep if given the opportunity?
    Probe: Do you find it easy to fall asleep? Can you stay asleep? After the baby is fed can you go back to sleep?

12. Do you have an appetite? When did you last eat? What have you eaten today? What's available to eat in your house?

13. Is there anybody in your family or a neighbor or friend who can watch the baby or help around the house?

14. Is there anybody you can talk to honestly about what you are experiencing?

If the parent is displaying moderate to severe symptoms of PPD, talk with the family to come up with a plan of action on how to help. Remember that the partner and other family members may also be having signs and symptoms of depression.

Handout 3

How to
help cope
with **PPD**

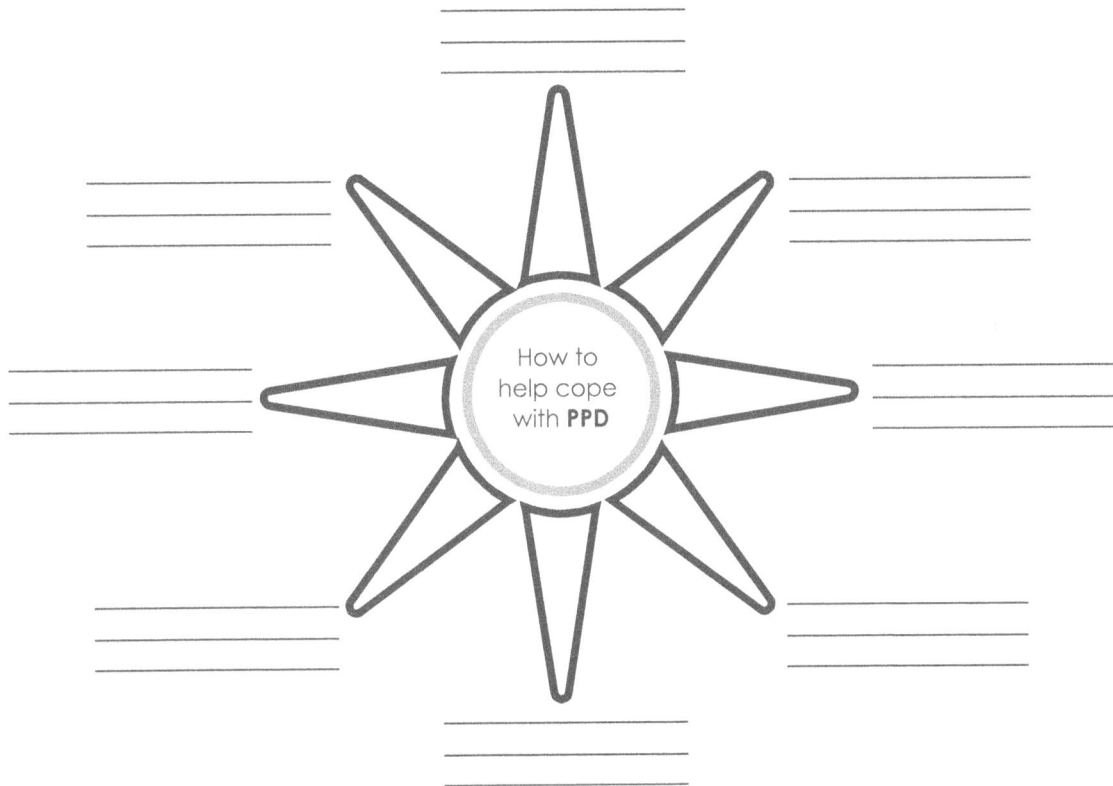

Universal Message:

1. You are not alone.

2. You are not to blame for what you are feeling.

3. You will be well and feel like yourself again.

Steps to Wellness:

Education about PPD: It is important that everyone knows about the onset, intensity, and duration of the signs and symptoms of PPD.

Sleep: Recovery depends on quality of sleep. Sleep can heal the body and mind. Someone not sleeping well may be suffering from depression or anxiety.

Eating nutritious food: If parents are not eating well, no one will thrive—including the baby.

Exercise and time for oneself: To be healthy the body requires a balance of sleep, food, and movement.

Nonjudgmental listening from others: New parents need to talk about their journey through pregnancy, birth or the adoption process, and parenthood.

Emotional support from others: New parents need supportive and caring people with whom to share and be heard.

Practical support from others: Parents need help.

Plan of Action:

Now let's make a plan of actions:

- How can you get more sleep?

- How is your appetite?

- Who can you ask for help?

- Who can you talk to about what you are experiencing

The components of *Steps to Wellness* work for everyone, not just new parents. All family members, including children, will benefit from these practical suggestions.

Handout 4

Peer support should strive to:

- Address the needs of at-risk populations.
  (women of reproductive age, parents-to-be, new parents, new grandparents)

- Confront social isolation.

- Serve as new sources of social support during short-term crises and life transitions.

- Promote coping skills and self-esteem.

- Provide positive role models.

- Display benefits of helping others.

- Meet needs of under-served portions of the population.

- Facilitate referrals to professionals when necessary.

- Enhance social ties to serve as a buffer to stress.

- Help people cope with stress and adversity.

- Educate professionals about gaps and problems in service delivery.

- Assist in development of needed programming for communities.

- Promote social action and funding needs.

- Promote new collaboration between self-help and professional communities.

Create a vision diagram:

1. Think about the current situation for new families in your community.

2. What support do new parents receive?

3. Imagine a future in which new parents and families are fully supported.

4. What would your role in this vision of the future be? What other roles might exist?

Handout 5

Evaluation of the Postpartum Action Workshop

Did this workshop meet the following goals and objectives?

Workshop Goals:

1. To reach and teach parents to be peer leaders

2. To have participants feel comfortable about the topic of depression

3. To learn and practice how to empower parents, their families, and others

Workshop Objectives:

1. Learned about postpartum depression (PPD)

2. Learned how to provide quality, personalized support for women and men experiencing PPD

3. Learned the "Steps to Wellness" that can help empower people to help themselves

4. Learned how to help individuals create a plan of action to help them assess their strengths and needs

5. Learned how to build a supportive community for families experiencing PPD

Use the space below and the back, if needed, to write your comments. Your feedback is appreciated.

SOURCES

Session 2, pages 19-20

Selim, N. "Cultural Dimensions of Depression in Bangladesh: A Qualitative Study in Two Villages of Matlab." *Journal of Health, Population, & Nutrition,* 2010. International Centre for Diarrhoeal Disease Research, Bangladesh.

Session 3, pages 21-23

The Centers for Disease Control and Prevention: *http://www.cdc.gov/reproductivehealth/Depression/*

Postpartum Education for Parents: *http://www.sbpep.org/ppd/*

Session 4, pages 25-27

"Tools Together Now! 100 Participatory Tools to Mobilize Communities for HIV/ AIDS." *International HIV/AIDS Alliance,* 2006. *http://www.aidsalliance.org/includes/ Publication/Tools_Together_Now_2009.pdf*

Session 5, pages 29-30

Honikman, Jane. *I'm Listening: A Guide to Supporting Postpartum Families,* 2024. *Amazon.com*

Session 6, pages 31-32

Trials of Improved Practice (TIPS): Guiding Notes for TIPS Trainers and Implementers. Food and Agriculture Organization of the United Nations (FAO), 2011. *http://www.fao.org/docrep/014/am868e/am868e00.pdf*

Session 7, pages 33-34

Madara, E.J. "Maximizing the Potential for Community Self-help Through Clearinghouse Approaches." *Prevention in Human Services,* 1990.

"Tools Together Now! 100 Participatory Tools to Mobilize Communities for HIV/AIDS." *International HIV/AIDS Alliance, 2006. http://www.aidsalliance.org/includes/Publication/Tools_ Together_Now_2009.pdf*

Honikman, Jane. *Community Support for New Families, 2013. Amazon.com*